Pocket Healing Books

Color
Healing

Barbara White

GW00778360

Astrolog Publishing House

Pocket Healing Books

Holistic Healing
Dr. Ilona Melman

Aromatherapy
Kevin Hudson

Reiki
Chantal Dupont

Vitamins
Jon Tillman

Bach Flowers
Susan Holden

Herbal Remedies
Dan Wolf

Minerals
Jon Tillman

Color Healing
Barbara White

Color healing

In ancient times, long before people knew anything about the body's systems, blood circulation, cells, muscle tissue, bones, or metabolism, they knew that the body transmitted various signals to its surface in order to signal a disease or a disorder.

The human body consists of a combination of the four elements: earth, fire, water, and air. It represents the elements in exactly the same way as the universe represents the elements. The glue that binds the elements together into "man" is harmonious equilibrium that obeys the laws of the universe.

When the body is in harmony with the divine order, the person is healthy. When the divine harmony in the body is disrupted, the person becomes ill.

In ancient times, the causes of diseases, bacteria, and so on were unknown. People considered the body to be a balanced system, and +evil spirits as enemies or assassins. Therefore, an evil spirit that invaded the body could well cause death.

Since many of the body's signals attesting to an "evil spirit" inside it entailed a change in its color, or in part of it, people considered color to be linked to the disruption of harmony. Colors such as red, yellow, black, white, purple, blue, and so on, appear on the body as the adjuncts of inflammations, blows, diseases, etc.

Since **the body signals by means of colors**, the battle against the evil spirit must be waged with colors! Thus we find a detailed key to the colors that are used in healing - or in the battle against the evil spirit that undermines the divine harmony - in rituals, amulets, and natural cures from former times.

When the evil spirit enters the body and disrupts its equilibrium, it secretes its toxic secretions, which can occur in various colors - each color causing a different disease.

Each kind of colored secretion, therefore, is counteracted by a healing color!

In the Germanic tribes of about two millennia ago, it was believed that the secretions of evil spirits came in nine colors. As an antidote, the person carried a rope woven from nine fibers or cords, each one in a different color (corresponding to the nine colors of the evil spirit's secretions).

This amulet protects against: "... the nine evil spirits, the nine colors of the secretions, and the nine winged diseases (that is, that are brought by the evil spirit, which has the ability to fly."

Since the color cures the disease, people looked for the medications themselves in the color phenomena on the face of the earth, in the aspects of nature with which they were familiar. One of the primary sources of color is plants, many of which became **herbal remedies** in ancient times, and plant essences in modern times.

When plants were used, many were found - through trial and error - to actually contain healing properties. However, their primary use lay in their colors.

Disease causes color - color cures disease!

This is the sharp, clear, and simple context for understanding color in healing.

In order to "bring" the effect of color to the body, and to expel the harmful evil spirit, people used plants, especially flowers, minerals (precious stones and crystals, mainly) and color essences that were extracted in various ways.

Many researchers and practitioners who try to find a way or method of healing by means of the properties of color, or of investigating healing by means of the laws of color, still consult Edwin D. Babbitt's book, which was published in 1878!

Babbitt, a well-known mystic, healer, and man of science of his time, published a book called "The Principles of Light and Color," and subtitled, "The Harmonic Laws of the Universe, the Etherio-Atomic Philosophy, Chromo Therapeutics, and the General Philosophy of Fine Forces, together with Numerous Discoveries and Practical Applications" - a long and clumsy title that did not prevent the book from becoming a basic text, and its author from being heralded as the prophet of color, the mystic who preceded his time - "the Jules Verne of the mysticism of color."

Even though Babbitt's book was used by many of his students and followers, it disappeared from the book market until the early seventies of the twentieth century. Now his book is being reprinted, albeit with a certain amount of editing. (The editions that were edited by David Ciranex, a mystic and healer in his own right, are the most faithful to the original. Regretfully, however, there are many editions that attempt to fix up and improve Babbitt's writings.)

Edwin D. Babbitt was born in 1828. His father was a church functionary. Edwin received a good education, and undertook many journeys in the Americas and abroad. He married at age 30, and had five children. For a living, he sold equipment to schools, including learning aids and books, some of which he printed himself.

In approximately 1870, Babbitt began to take an interest in the fields of mysticism and metaphysics, especially in the metaphysical field of magnetism and healing by means of magnetic energy. As a result of his studies, he became involved in active magnetic healing, and began to formulate the principles of his color theory.

At that time, anyone could practice healing or medicine, and Babbitt was considered by many as nothing more than a charlatan who earned his living by magnetic or color healing, in the same way as others sold miracle drugs or healing stones! However, whoever came across Babbitt's well-known book and read it was immediately won over by the systematic nature of his method, by the broad spectrum he covered, and by the apparently simple principles upon which his world of colors was based.

Babbitt died in 1905, without seeing his theory becoming common knowledge. Only decades after his death was his theory given due credit in the field of mysticism and color healing.

It is important to remember that in his time, Babbitt was not the only one seeking a spiritual-physical cure by means of color. For instance, many people sought wonder drugs in the "sky" - a combination of blue and yellow, colors that afforded the requisite power for creating life. In this field, for example, there were people who erected hothouses that were painted blue, claiming that the fruits and vegetables grown in them were more healthful, and had great "natural powers," because of the effect of the color blue and the yellow rays of the sun. (In New York, this method was an outcome of the Dutch settlement, since the Dutch had painted the interior walls of barns, cow-sheds, and hothouses blue for generations, in the belief that it eliminated pests and insects.)

Other people tried to develop entire theories

based on the colors blue and red, and their effect on people's health. "White light receives the moving color blue and the stable color black on the negative pole; while on the positive pole, it passes from moving yellow to fixed red. Blue invites action, black causes stagnation (death); yellow is active, red is the movement of life. **Therefore, white is the balance of the healthy movement.**"

Or, in another version, "Red is the climax of man's life, and from there the path descends the slope until it reaches the black end ... white is the active path along which man goes from stage to stage in his life..."

These theories led to the development of healing instruments - colored lenses that filtered light. The explanation in the brochure that came with the set of color lenses for self-healing read as follows: "In order to accelerate and strengthen the nervous system, use a red filter ... in order to calm down the body system, use a blue filter, and in this way you will avoid tension and nervousness."

Babbitt was well acquainted with the color healers of his time - and his big advantage lay in his ability to make his theory more profound, to combine it with scientific knowledge - mainly the movement of atoms, or the energy **within** the color atom - and with the historical knowledge he had accumulated about spiritual and physical color healing (in his library, there were about 4,000 books pertaining to one or other aspect of the history of color healing).

The entire theory propounded by Babbitt was the one that placed him head and shoulders above the other color healers - Plissenton, Fanstock, Barley, or Goldwyn, who were his contemporaries and were very famous. **Babbitt was the only one who propounded an entire theory that can be tested and applied nowadays as well!**

Babbitt analyzed the cases he treated, and provided general instructions. A treatment ("a bath of colored radiation," as he called it) with the color red cures conditions of spiritual and physical exhaustion, paralysis, and nervous depression; a treatment with yellow or orange charges the person with energy for everyday life; yellow alone cures respiratory ailments; yellow with red repairs the desires of the flesh (in other words, improves sexuality); blue and purple solve problems of the nervous system, migraines, allergies, and so on.

In addition to the unique treatment, Babbitt also tried to give "preventive treatment" in order to safeguard the spiritual and physical health of the average person. To do this, Babbitt researched many Christian historical sources and discovered, for instance, that in many churches there were pieces of colored glass in the windows (stained glass windows). The colors of the glass and the combination of colors induced a particular atmosphere in each church. Babbitt maintained that the special atmosphere in each church was the result of the multicolored windows that were unique to it.

From the point of view of healing, the fact that Babbitt penetrated Western consciousness with the subject of natural light is very important. Until his time, sunlight - natural light - was considered harmful to health. Babbitt taught people that exposure to sunlight prevented diseases and cured other diseases. (We must remember that Babbitt worked in regions in which the danger of excessive sunshine did not exist - England or North America, for instance.) He taught people to forgo their sunshades, closed carriages, or full-length bathing suits. Babbitt recommended that sick people expose their bodies to sunlight. He particularly recommended this for pregnant woman and for mothers of infants - on condition that they take their babies with them into the sunlight (sunlight improves the quality of mother's milk); and for people who were in the "twilight" of their lives - at his time, this meant people of fifty and over.

How is color used?

This simple question conceals countless answers. The easiest answer is - however you like! And this is not just being facetious.

The general division is made according to five principal methods:

1. By taking color into the body. This is done by drinking a colored beverage - in the form of drops of essences and so on - or drinking water in which various crystals of appropriate colors have been immersed.

2. By projecting light through colored glass or a transparent material painted in the appropriate color, like Babbitt's fundamental principle - a colored window that projects light.

3. By focusing the vision on a colored surface - this method is good for short periods of time, and must be accompanied by thoughts about the color.

4. By spending time in an appropriate environment - for instance, a hike through a green forest, or being in yellow sand, and so on.

5. By activating the consciousness, and subconsciously linking up to the appropriate color.

Let's suppose that you want to focus on the color blue for an hour a day.

You could place a blue crystal in a glass of water overnight, and sip the water slowly over the course of an hour. (Make sure that the crystal is suitable for preparing a potion.)

You can spend an hour staring at a sheet of blue paper.

You can spend time in a room that is mostly (at least 80 percent) shades of blue.

You can paint a light-bulb blue and turn on the light, and so on.

Every person must find the method that suits him the best. Several methods can be used, switching methods each time.

Experienced practitioners use bottles of color (which contain liquids that are not potable!) that they carry with them, place on a table next to their beds, and so on.

The highest stage of the use of color - by the consciousness - is a relatively difficult stage, which only a few people reach.

Index for Treating Diseases

The names of the diseases are arranged in alphabetical order. They are general names, and are based more on symptoms than on medical diagnoses. If a particular disease is not mentioned, look for **similar characteristics** (shortness of breath - asthma, for example). You can use the principle of "similarity" - for instance, learn about a hair treatment from "Hair loss," and so on. An asterisk (*) indicates that the disease has its own entry.

Acne
Preferred treatment: Green
Possible treatment: Blue and yellow
Length of time: Ten minutes a day
Colors to avoid: Mainly red and magenta

Airsickness
Preferred treatment: White
Possible treatment: Yellow
Length of time: As long as necessary
Colors to avoid: Mainly blue and green

Alcoholism
Preferred treatment: Orange
Possible treatment: Turquoise
Length of time: Thirty minutes each morning
Colors to avoid: Mainly red and blue

Allergies
Preferred treatment: Green
Possible treatment: Brown and yellow together
Length of time: Unlimited
Color to avoid: Mainly magenta

Amenorrhea (failure to menstruate)
Preferred treatment: White
Possible treatment: Yellow
Length of time: Five minutes, six times a day
Color to avoid: Mainly red

Anal itching
Preferred treatment: Brown
Possible treatment: Silver
Length of time: Five minutes every two hours
Colors to avoid: Mainly red and magenta

Anemia
Preferred treatment: Red
Possible treatment: Orange
Length of time: Unlimited
Color to avoid: Mainly purple

Anorexia
Preferred treatment: White
Possible treatment: Green
Length of time: Ten minutes, before every meal
Color to avoid: Mainly black

Apathy, listlessness
Preferred treatment: White (clear light)
Possible treatment: Green
Length of time: Unlimited
Colors to avoid: Mainly black and brown

Arrhythmia (irregular heartbeat)
Preferred treatment: Blue
Possible treatment: Green
Length of time: An hour a day
Color to avoid: Mainly yellow

Arteriosclerosis
Preferred treatment: Red
Possible treatment: Magenta
Length of time: Ten minutes twice a day

Colors to avoid: Mainly blue and green
Arthritis
Preferred treatment: Brown or black
Possible treatment: Gray
Length of time: An hour a day
Color to avoid: Mainly white

Asthma
Preferred treatment: A combination of green, yellow and blue
Possible treatment: Yellow alone
Length of time: Ten minutes every hour for an entire week
Color to avoid: Mainly brown

Balding, premature balding
Preferred treatment: Red
Possible treatment: Magenta
Length of time: Ten minutes every hour for two consecutive weeks
Color to avoid: Mainly yellow

Bedwetting
Preferred treatment: Yellow
Possible treatment: White
Length of time: Thirty minutes every evening
Color to avoid: Mainly red

Benign tumor
Preferred treatment: As for Malignant tumor*, but no more than two hours a day.

Bleeding gums
Preferred treatment: Red
Possible treatment: Magenta
Length of time: As long as necessary
Color to avoid: Mainly white

Blocked gall ducts
Preferred treatment: Green
Possible treatment: Green with yellow
Length of time: As long as necessary
Color to avoid: Mainly red

Blood vessel diseases
Preferred treatment: Red
Possible treatment: Magenta
Length of time: Ten minutes a day
Color to avoid: Mainly black

Blurred vision
Preferred treatment: Black
Possible treatment: None
Length of time: Thirty minutes at noon
Color to avoid: Mainly white

Boils
Preferred treatment: Yellow
Possible treatment: Green
Length of time: Until healed
Color to avoid: Mainly red

Brittle bones
Preferred treatment: Red
Possible treatment: Purple
Length of time: As long as necessary, continuously
Color to avoid: Mainly white **or** black

Bronchial asthma - as for Asthma*

Bronchitis
Preferred treatment: Green
Possible treatment: Yellow
Length of time: Unlimited
Color to avoid: Mainly brown

Burns
Preferred treatment: Red
Possible treatment: Purple
Length of time: As long as necessary, continuously
Color to avoid: Mainly green

Cataract - as for Eye disorders*

Cessation of menstruation
Preferred treatment: Red
Possible treatment: Magenta
Length of time: Ten minutes once a day
Color to avoid: Mainly white

Cessation of urination
Preferred treatment: Yellow
Possible treatment: White
Length of time: Ten minutes every morning
Color to avoid: Mainly red

Chest pains
Preferred treatment: Green
Possible treatment: Turquoise
Length of time: As long as necessary
Colors to avoid: Mainly red and purple

Cholera
Preferred treatment: Yellow
Possible treatment: White
Length of time: An hour a day
Color to avoid: Mainly green

Colds
Preferred treatment: Green
Possible treatment: Red (for chronic colds)
Length of time: Unlimited time during the cold
Colors to avoid: Mainly yellow and white

Cold sores
Preferred treatment: White
Possible treatment: Yellow
Length of time: As long as necessary
Color to avoid: Mainly black

Colitis (inflammation of the large intestine) - as for Digestive disorders*

Conjunctivitis
Preferred treatment: Blue
Possible treatment: Purple
Length of time: Ten minutes every two hours
Color to avoid: Mainly yellow
Constipation - as for Digestive disorders*

Cramps
Preferred treatment: Magenta
Possible treatment: Red
Length of time: As long as necessary
Color to avoid: Mainly yellow

Cramps in the leg muscles
Preferred treatment: As for Cramps*, but with breaks of an hour between each time.

Cysts
Preferred treatment: Green
Possible treatment: Blue
Length of time: Ten minutes, three times a day
Color to avoid: Mainly red

Dandruff - as for Hair loss*, continuously for a week

Deafness
Preferred treatment: Brown
Possible treatment: Purple, black
Length of time: Ten minutes every morning
Color to avoid: Mainly blue

Defective muscle power
Preferred treatment: Red
Possible treatment: Magenta
Length of time: Thirty minutes a day
Color to avoid: Mainly black

Dehydration
Preferred treatment: Yellow
Possible treatment: White
Length of time: A full hour
Color to avoid: Mainly black

Diabetes
Preferred treatment: Red
Possible treatment: Magenta
Length of time: Unlimited, **continuous**
Color to avoid: Mainly green

Diarrhea - as for Digestive disorders*

Digestive disorders
Preferred treatment: Red
Possible treatment: Brown
Length of time: As long as necessary
Color to avoid: Mainly green

Diseases accompanied by a high fever
Preferred treatment: Green
Possible treatment: Blue
Length of time: As long as necessary
Color to avoid: Mainly red

Dislocated shoulder - as for Muscle tension*

Drop in energy
Preferred treatment: Red
Possible treatment: Red combined with purple
Length of time: Unlimited
Colors to avoid: Mainly black and brown

Dryness in the nasal membranes
Preferred treatment: Green
Possible treatment: Blue combined with yellow
Length of time: Unlimited
Color to avoid: Mainly red

Dysgraphia as a result of a cerebral defect
Preferred treatment: Purple
Possible treatment: Blue
Length of time: Thirty minutes once a week
Color to avoid: Mainly gray

Earache
Preferred treatment: Green
Possible treatment: Green combined with yellow
Length of time: As long as necessary
Color to avoid: Mainly red

Eczema
Preferred treatment: Green
Possible treatment: Blue and yellow
Length of time: Unlimited
Colors to avoid: Mainly red and magenta

Edema
Preferred treatment: Blue
Possible treatment: Turquoise
Length of time: Five minutes every two hours
Color to avoid: Mainly yellow

Epileptic attack
Preferred treatment: Brown
Possible treatment: Black
Length of time: As long as necessary
Color to avoid: Mainly white

Excessive perspiration
Preferred treatment: Green
Possible treatment: Black
Length of time: Thirty minutes every morning
Colors to avoid: Mainly yellow, gold, and white

Eye disorders, including far- and near-sightedness, glaucoma, astigmatism, and aging of the eye
Preferred treatment: Green
Possible treatment: Blue
Length of time: Unlimited
Color to avoid: Mainly yellow

Food poisoning
Preferred treatment: Green
Possible treatment: Green combined with blue
Length of time: An entire day
Color to avoid: Mainly red

Functional problems as a result of a stroke
Preferred treatment: Red
Possible treatment: Purple
Length of time: Unlimited
Color to avoid: Mainly yellow

Gallstones
Preferred treatment: Green
Possible treatment: Yellow and blue together
Length of time: Ten minutes, twice a day
Colors to avoid: Mainly magenta and red

Gas in the stomach or intestines
Preferred treatment: Yellow
Possible treatment: Orange
Length of time: Up to three hours
Colors to avoid: Mainly green and blue

General itching
Preferred treatment: Brown
Possible treatment: Silver
Length of time: Unlimited
Color to avoid: Mainly red

Hair loss
Preferred treatment: Purple
Possible treatment: Red
Length of time: Three months without a break
Colors to avoid: Mainly black, brown, and gray

Hayfever - as for Asthma*

Headache
Preferred treatment: Green
Possible treatment: Green with the addition of blue
Length of time: As long as necessary
Color to avoid: Mainly red

Heart attack
Preferred treatment: Green
Possible treatment: Light blue
Length of time: Unlimited
Color to avoid: Mainly red

Heartburn
Preferred treatment: Blue
Possible treatment: Turquoise
Length of time: As long as necessary
Color to avoid: Mainly red

Hemorrhoids
Preferred treatment: Red
Possible treatment: Magenta
Length of time: Twenty minutes every day
Colors to avoid: Mainly brown and black

Hepatitis
Preferred treatment: Purple
Possible treatment: Magenta
Length of time: As long as necessary
Colors to avoid: Mainly yellow and green

Hernia
Preferred treatment: White
Possible treatment: None
Length of time: Continuously until problem is solved
Colors to avoid: Mainly dark colors

Herpes simplex
Preferred treatment: Red
Possible treatment: Magenta
Length of time: Unlimited
Color to avoid: Mainly white

Hiccups, belching
Preferred treatment: White
Possible treatment: Yellow
Length of time: As long as necessary
Color to avoid: Mainly red

High / low blood pressure
Preferred treatment: Green
Possible treatment: Blue
Length of time: Unlimited
Color to avoid: Mainly red

Hoarseness
Preferred treatment: Brown
Possible treatment: Red
Length of time: Ten minutes
Colors to avoid: Mainly green, blue

Hot flashes
Preferred treatment: Blue
Possible treatment: Turquoise
Length of time: Up to six hours a day
Colors to avoid: Orange and red

Hyperexcitability
Preferred treatment: Green
Possible treatment: Turquoise
Length of time: As long as necessary
Color to avoid: Mainly red

Hypertension
Preferred treatment: Green
Possible treatment: Blue
Length of time: Unlimited
Color to avoid: Mainly red

Hysteria
Preferred treatment: Turquoise
Possible treatment: Blue
Length of time: Unlimited
Color to avoid: Mainly purple

Impotence
Preferred treatment: Red
Possible treatment: White
Length of time: Fifteen minutes twice a day
Colors to avoid: Mainly green, blue + yellow, purple

Infection
Preferred treatment: Red
Possible treatment: Blue
Length of time: Ten minutes a day
Color to avoid: Mainly brown

Infertility
Preferred treatment: Red
Possible treatment: Magenta
Length of time: Half a year, continuously
Color to avoid: Mainly yellow

Inflammations
Preferred treatment: Red
Possible treatment: Orange
Length of time: Ten minutes a day
Color to avoid: Mainly brown

Inflammation of the ankle bone -
see Inflammations*

Inflammation of the bladder
Preferred treatment: Yellow
Possible treatment: Gold
Length of time: Ten minutes a day
Color to avoid: Mainly black

Inflammation of the eyelids -
see Conjunctivitis*

Inflammation of the fallopian tubes -
see Inflammations*

Inflammation of the gall bladder -
see Inflammations*

Inflammation of the gall ducts -
see Inflammations*

Inflammation of the larynx / soft palate -
see Inflammations*

Inflammation of the large intestine
Preferred treatment: Red
Possible treatment: Orange
Length of time: Unlimited
Color to avoid: Mainly brown

Inflammation of the liver -
see Inflammations*

Inflammation of the ovary -
see Inflammations*

Inflammation of the prostate -
see Inflammations*

Inflammation of the shoulder joint -
see Inflammations*

Inflammation of the stomach
Preferred treatment: As for Inflammation of the large intestine*, but not longer than three consecutive hours

Inflammation of the stomach muscles -
see Inflammations*

Inflammation of the throat -
see Inflammations*

Inflammation of the uterus -
see Inflammations*

Inflammation of the wrist joint -
see Inflammations*

Influenza - as for Asthma*, continuously

Insanity
Preferred treatment: Green
Possible treatment: Blue
Length of time: Unlimited
Color to avoid: Mainly purple
Insomnia - as for Migraine*, before going to sleep

Irregular periods
Preferred treatment: Red
Possible treatment: Red combined with purple
Length of time: Thirty minutes a day for two consecutive days
Color to avoid: Mainly green

Lack of blood cell production
Preferred treatment: Red
Possible treatment: Red with magenta
Length of time: Unlimited
Color to avoid: Mainly green

Lack of milk
Preferred treatment: Green
Possible treatment: Yellow and blue
Length of time: Unlimited
Colors to avoid: A combination of more than three colors

Lack of self-control / nervous problems
Preferred treatment: Green
Possible treatment: Blue + yellow
Length of time: Unlimited
Color to avoid: Mainly red

Lack of virility / absence of erection
Preferred treatment: Purple
Possible treatment: Red
Length of time: Thirty minutes a day
Color to avoid: Mainly white

Loss of balance
Preferred treatment: Red
Possible treatment: Purple or magenta
Length of time: Two hours
Color to avoid: Mainly turquoise

Loss of consciousness
Preferred treatment: Red
Possible treatment: Purple
Length of time: Until consciousness is regained
Color to avoid: Mainly black

Low sperm count
Preferred treatment: White
Possible treatment: Purple, red
Length of time: Up to two hours a day
Color to avoid: Mainly black

Lymph gland diseases
Preferred treatment: Yellow
Possible treatment: White
Length of time: Unlimited
Colors to avoid: Mainly black and brown

Malignant tumor
Preferred treatment: Green
Possible treatment: None
Length of time: Unlimited
Color to avoid: Mainly red

Massive hemorrhage / stroke
Preferred treatment: Red
Possible treatment: Magenta
Length of time: As long as necessary
Color to avoid: Mainly white

Measles
Preferred treatment: Red
Possible treatment: Red and magenta
Length of time: The duration of the disease
Colors to avoid: Mainly yellow and white

Meningitis - see Inflammations*

Mental disturbances
Preferred treatment: Green combined with blue
Possible treatment: Light blue
Length of time: Unlimited
Color to avoid: Mainly red

Mental unrest
Preferred treatment: Green
Possible treatment: Blue
Length of time: An hour a day
Colors to avoid: Mainly purple and black

Migraine
Preferred treatment: Green
Possible treatment: Blue
Length of time: Thirty minutes when necessary
Color to avoid: Mainly purple

Miscarriage
Preferred treatment: Green
Possible treatment: Blue
Length of time: Six consecutive hours, every day
Color to avoid: Mainly purple

Muscle degeneration
Preferred treatment: Red
Possible treatment: Purple
Length of time: An hour a day, in the morning
Color to avoid: Mainly yellow

Muscle tension
Preferred treatment: Green
Possible treatment: Blue
Length of time: Ten minutes when necessary
Color to avoid: Mainly red

Nausea
Preferred treatment: Yellow
Possible treatment: Gold
Length of time: As long as necessary
Color to avoid: Mainly blue

Neck pains - as for Chest pains*

Nervousness
Preferred treatment: Green
Possible treatment: Blue with yellow
Length of time: As long as necessary, every day
Color to avoid: Mainly red

Nervous tics
Preferred treatment: Green
Possible treatment: Brown
Length of time: Unlimited, **continuous**
Colors to avoid: Mainly white and yellow

Nightmares
Preferred treatment: Green
Possible treatment: Blue
Length of time: An hour, before going to sleep
Color to avoid: Mainly black

Night sweats
Preferred treatment: As for Excessive perspiration*, but only ten minutes twice a day.

Non-salivation
Preferred treatment: Green
Possible treatment: Blue or yellow
Length of time: Ten minutes a day
Color to avoid: Mainly brown

Nosebleed
Preferred treatment: Red
Possible treatment: None
Length of time: As long as necessary
Color to avoid: Mainly white

Obesity
Preferred treatment: White
Possible treatment: Yellow
Length of time: Unlimited
Color to avoid: Mainly black

Obsession
Preferred treatment: Yellow
Possible treatment: Gold, white
Length of time: Two hours every two days
Colors to avoid: Mainly black, brown, and purple

Pain (general)
Preferred treatment: Green
Possible treatment: Blue
Length of time: Unlimited
Colors to avoid: Mainly red and black

Pain in the Achilles tendon, in the thigh muscle, in the nerves of the leg
Preferred treatment: Blue
Possible treatment: Green
Length of time: Thirty minutes a day
Color to avoid: Mainly brown

Pain in the arms
Preferred treatment: Green
Possible treatment: Orange (with extreme caution!)
Length of time: Thirty minutes
Color to avoid: Mainly black

Pain in the back, hips, and shoulder-blades
Preferred treatment: Green
Possible treatment: Blue
Length of time: As long as necessary
Colors to avoid: Mainly black and white

Pain in the bones - as for Pain (general)*, one hour a day

Pain in the eyes - as for Blurred vision*, unlimited time, as necessary

Pain in the kidneys
Preferred treatment: Red
Possible treatment: Magenta
Length of time: Thirty minutes a day
Colors to avoid: Mainly blue and green

Pain in the ovaries
Preferred treatment: Green
Possible treatment: Red (with extreme caution!)
Length of time: Ten minutes a day
Colors to avoid: Mainly brown and orange

Pain in the thigh, the foot, the heel
Preferred treatment: Blue
Possible treatment: Green
Length of time: Ten minutes a day
Colors to avoid: Mainly brown and black

Pains during urination
Preferred treatment: Yellow
Possible treatment: Orange
Length of time: As long as necessary
Color to avoid: Mainly red

Pains in the breast
Preferred treatment: Green
Possible treatment: Blue
Length of time: As long as necessary
Color to avoid: Mainly black

Pains in the nape of the neck - see Pain in the back*

Paralysis of the diaphragm
Preferred treatment: Yellow
Possible treatment: White
Length of time: As long as necessary
Color to avoid: Mainly black

Phobias, panic
Preferred treatment: White
Possible treatment: Yellow, silver
Length of time: As long as necessary
Color to avoid: Mainly black

Pins and needles in the foot or hand
Preferred treatment: Green
Possible treatment: Green with the addition of blue
Length of time: As long as necessary
Color to avoid: Mainly red

Pneumonia
Preferred treatment: Green
Possible treatment: Turquoise
Length of time: Unlimited
Color to avoid: Mainly red

Premenstrual tension
Preferred treatment: Blue
Possible treatment: Green
Length of time: As long as necessary
Color to avoid: Mainly red

Quitting smoking
Preferred treatment: White
Possible treatment: Green
Length of time: Ten minutes every hour, during daylight, for a whole week
Color to avoid: Mainly black

Rapid heartbeat
Preferred treatment: Blue
Possible treatment: Green
Length of time: As long as necessary
Color to avoid: Mainly red

Respiratory disturbances
Preferred treatment: Green
Possible treatment: Blue
Length of time: Ten minutes every hour, when needed
Colors to avoid: Mainly brown and black

Runny nose
Preferred treatment: Green
Possible treatment: Yellow
Length of time: As long as necessary
Color to avoid: Mainly red

Seasickness - see Airsickness*

Shock
Preferred treatment: Red
Possible treatment: Magenta
Length of time: Unlimited
Color to avoid: Mainly green

Shortness of breath - see Asthma*

Sinusitis
Preferred treatment: Green
Possible treatment: Yellow
Length of time: An hour every morning for two weeks
Colors to avoid: Mainly red and black

Skin (general problems)
Preferred treatment: Green
Possible treatment: Yellow, red
Length of time: Up to two hours a day
Color to avoid: Mainly black

Slow heartbeat
Preferred treatment: Red
Possible treatment: Purple
Length of time: Thirty minutes once a day
Color to avoid: Mainly black

Slowness/procrastination
Preferred treatment: Blue
Possible treatment: Purple or yellow
Length of time: Unlimited
Color to avoid: Mainly magenta

Sores
Preferred treatment: Red
Possible treatment: Yellow, green
Length of time: Until healed
Color to avoid: Mainly white

Sore throat
Preferred treatment: Green
Possible treatment: Blue
Length of time: Ten minutes twice a day
Color to avoid: Mainly brown

Speech impediment
Preferred treatment: Blue
Possible treatment: Turquoise
Length of time: Ten minutes twice a day
Color to avoid: Mainly white

Stiff back
Preferred treatment: Orange
Possible treatment: Magenta
Length of time: Twenty minutes once a day
Colors to avoid: Mainly green and blue

Stiff knee
Preferred treatment: Turquoise
Possible treatment: Blue
Length of time: Unlimited
Colors to avoid: Mainly red and orange

Stiff neck - as for Stiff back*, but with unlimited time

Stomach-ache
Preferred treatment: Green
Possible treatment: Blue
Length of time: As long as necessary
Color to avoid: Mainly red

Stomach ulcer
Preferred treatment: White
Possible treatment: Yellow
Length of time: Thirty minutes a day
Colors to avoid: Mainly green and blue

Stuffy nose
Preferred treatment: A combination of the
treatments for asthma* and bronchitis*

Stuttering
Preferred treatment: Purple
Possible treatment: Red
Length of time: Ten minutes a day
Color to avoid: Mainly yellow

Sunstroke
Preferred treatment: Blue
Possible treatment: Red
Length of time: As long as necessary
Color to avoid: Mainly black

Toothache
Preferred treatment: White
Possible treatment: Green
Length of time: As long as necessary
Color to avoid: Mainly black

Varicosis
Preferred treatment: Magenta
Possible treatment: White
Length of time: Thirty minutes every two days
Color to avoid: Mainly green

Vertigo
Preferred treatment: Green
Possible treatment: Brown
Length of time: As long as necessary
Color to avoid: Mainly white

Vomiting
Preferred treatment: Green
Possible treatment: Blue and yellow
Length of time: Twenty minutes every morning for a week
Colors to avoid: Mainly brown and black

Weak heart muscle
Preferred treatment: Green and red in equal proportions
Possible treatment: Red alone
Length of time: Up to an entire week
Color to avoid: Mainly black

Weakness
Preferred treatment: Green
Possible treatment: Green combined with turquoise
Length of time: Unlimited
Color to avoid: Mainly black

Weak vision
Preferred treatment: Purple
Possible treatment: Red with magenta
Length of time: Thirty minutes a day
Color to avoid: Mainly yellow

Color environment for good health

We repeat the warning:
**The contents of this book do not constitute a recommendation for medical treatment, a medical prescription, or medical advice.
When there is a medical problem, an appropriate physician must be consulted.**

Color is not just meant for curing diseases or facilitating their cure. Color is an excellent means of **maintaining good health and preventing disease.**

Whatever the person's state of health, however old he is, and wherever he is situated, his physical health can be improved.

The case of an English prisoner, Patrick Quentin, was widely publicized in the British press in 1991.

Patrick Quentin was arrested, sentenced, and jailed for 12 years for committing armed robbery, during the course of which an innocent passer-by was killed. He was incarcerated in a facility that was controlled by a gang that had a score to settle with him. As a result, he was forced to live in a protected cell for most of his sentence.

Patrick Quentin's wife worked in a New Age store in London, and when she told her employer about her husband's predicament, the employer suggested that Patrick's cell be decorated with squares of color, according to a pattern that she gave her.

Although the suggestion initially met with ridicule, Patrick's cell was painted according to the design.

When Patrick was released from prison, it turned out that his state of health - both physical and mental - had improved amazingly, and was far better than that of other prisoners who had had access to the prison yard and engaged in daily physical exercise. Diseases that Patrick had had in the past, including serious intestinal ailments, disappeared. Although he had not engaged in any physical exercise, his muscles maintained their strength and flexible, and he looked "ten years younger than his actual age." There was also an improvement in his mental condition, and he became calm and tranquil, and kicked - as far as we know - the alcohol and drug habits without any formal rehabilitation framework.

Patrick Quentin appeared in several interviews, and as a result of his case, it was decided that prisoners' cells would be painted in color patterns that were carefully chosen by color healers. This experiment has not yet been completed, but there has already been a tremendous improvement in the condition of the inhabitants of the painted cells.

The British Institute for the [medical] Use of Color offers color coordination services to places such as schools, hospitals, offices, and stores. The color coordination does not aim to "stimulate" casual clients or customers, but is rather an expression of a sincere concern for the people who spend long hours every day working or studying in these places.

The cumulative results of approximately ten years of work appear in two charts that are meant for people who are healthy (in comparison with people of the same age) and do not suffer from any particular diseases. Table 1 (A and B) indicates the range of colors and the percentage of each color in the background of the person's surroundings, according to age and gender. Table 2 indicates the desired color composition during the various hours of the day - including the hours of artificial lighting (at night).

The colors are divided into seven colors only (blue includes turquoise, red includes magenta, and so on). The recommendationsallow up to five percent deviation in each color, but it must be remembered that when one color is decreased, another must be increased. Each color is given a minimum value (in the first line) and a maximum value (in the second line).

The colors that are taken into account are those in the **background** of the place where the person lives.

Everyone should examine his surroundings, and construct a color model according to his choice, so that he reaches at least 80 percent of his total range of colors.

For example: A 16-year-old girl

Yellow - 24, green - 30, red - 14, blue - 20.

Table 1A: Color Chart According to Gender and Age, in %

Women

Color	Up to 20 years old	Up to 35 years old	50 years and over
Purple	8 11	8 11	6 8
Red	14 20	12 17	10 14
Yellow	24 28	26 30	30 40
Orange	10 14	10 14	12 18
Green	30 40	25 33	22 29
Blue	20 25	20 25	20 25
Black	6 8	6 8	6 8

Table 1B: Color Chart According to Gender and Age, in %

Men

Color	Up to 20 years old	Up to 35 years old	50 years and over
Purple	6 9	6 9	5 7
Red	16 22	14 19	12 16
Yellow	24 28	26 30	30 40
Orange	5 7	5 7	6 9
Green	30 35	25 28	22 26
Blue	25 30	25 30	20 25
Black	6 12	6 12	6 12

Table 2: Recommended Colors According to the Hours of the Day

Dawn - Sunrise
Yellow, orange, and green

Morning
Green, blue

Noon
Blue, purple

Afternoon
Red, black (a little), blue

Evening
Red, yellow

Night (darkness)
Purple, yellow

Astrolog Publishing House
P. O. Box 1123, Hod Hasharon 45111, Israel
Tel: 972-9-7412044
Fax: 972-9-7442714
E-Mail: info@astrolog.co.il
Astrolog Web Site: www.astrolog.co.il

ISBN 965-494-116-3

Published by Astrolog Publishing House 2000

Printed in Israel
2 4 6 8 10 9 7 5 3 1